GASTROINTESTINAL REFLUX DISEASE (GERD) MANAGEMENT DIET COOKBOOK

Delicious Recipes And Lifestyle Tips For Acid Flow Back Relief:A Comprehensive Guide To Soothing Your Digestive System Naturally

DR. SHAYLA LEWIS

Table of Contents

CHAPTER ONE 14
   An explanation of acid reflux disease (GERD) 14
      Diet is Important for GERD Management 15
      Control Your Portion: 16
      Sustaining a Healthy Weight 16
      Meal Timing: 17
      Hydration: 17
      Low-Carb Diet: 18
      Antioxidant-Rich Diet: 18
      Anti-Inflammatory Diet 19
   Managing Neuropathy and Nerve Pain 19
   Planning Meals and Cooking in Bulk 20
      Managed Portions 20
      Balanced Nutrition 20
      Consistent Eating pattern: 21
      Cost-effective 21
CHAPTER TWO 22
   A Comprehensive Guide for Meal Planning: 22
      Make a Menu: 22

Make a Shopping List: 22

Prepare Ingredients: 23

Cook in Batches 23

Store Correctly..23

Recommendations for Busy People on Batch Cooking...23

Invest in Top-Rated Storage Containers 24

Use Kitchen Appliances 24

Rotate Meals: 24

Convenient Storage and Freezing Methods..25

Portion Control 25

Freeze Meals Correctly: 25

Use Freezer-Friendly items 25

Example Menus for Various Dietary Choices:...26

Low-Acid Dietary Schedule: 26

Meal Plan for Vegetarians: 26

Whole Wheat Meal Plan: 27

Chronic Acid Exposure: 28

Inflammation: 28

Side effects of medicine: 28

Nutritional Deficiencies: 29
Optimising GERD Treatment 29
Pain Management treatments: 29
Resolving Nutritional Deficiencies: 30
Stress Management: 30
CHAPTER THREE 32
Important elements of a GERD sufferer's healthy lifestyle include 32
   Dietary Modifications 32
   Frequent Exercise: 32
   Stress Management: 32
Diet is Important for GERD Management 34
   Important food factors for managing GERD include: 34
   Eating Slowly: 35
   Sustaining a Healthy Weight: 35
   Meal Timing: 36
   Hydration 36
   Low-Carb Diet: 37
   Antioxidant-Rich Diet: 37
   Anti-Inflammatory Diet: 38
Managing Neuropathy and Nerve Pain 38

Chronic Acid Exposure: 39

Side effects of medicine: 40

Nutritional Deficiencies: 40

Optimising GERD Treatment: 40

Pain Management treatments 41

Resolving Nutritional Deficiencies: 41

Stress Management: 41

Adopting a Healthful Lifestyle for Prolonged Well-Being 42

CHAPTER FOUR 44

Important elements of a GERD sufferer's healthy lifestyle include 44

    Dietary Modifications 44

    Frequent Exercise: 44

    Stress Management: 44

    Sleep Hygiene: 45

    Giving Up Smoking: 45

    Limiting Alcohol and Caffeine: 45

    Fundamentals of Nutrition. 46

    Macronutrients 46

    Micronutrients 47

    Fibre: 48

    Protein 49

Healthy Fats 49
Trigger Foods 50
Trigger Beverages 51
CHAPTER FIVE 52
Including Variation in a Balanced Diet 52
   Nutrient Diversity: 52
   Dietary Balance: 52
   Serving Size 53
   Nutrient Content 54
   Ingredients List: 54
   Living Low-Carb 55
   Non-Starchy Vegetables: 55
   Lean Proteins 56
   Good Fats 56
   Low-Sugar Fruits: 56
   Dairy: 56
Effective Blood Sugar Management 57
   Low-Carb Diets' Advantages for GERD 58
   Decreased Acid Reflux: 58
   Weight control: 58
   Improved Gut Health: 59
   Balanced Blood Sugar Levels 59

Yummy Low-Carb Recipes for Any Occasion 59

Snacks 60

Advice for Eating Out While Keeping Your Carbs Low 60

Ask for Modifications 61

Be Aware of Hidden Carbs: 61

Foods High in Antioxidants 62

CHAPTER SIX 64

Disease of Gastrointestinal Reflux (GERD) 64

GERD and Foods High in Antioxidants 64

Berries: 65

Leafy Greens 66

Nuts and Seeds 66

Brightly colored vegetables: 66

Herbs & Spices 66

Making Luminous and High-Nutrient Meals 66

How to Include Superfoods in Your Diet 67

Consuming Anti-Inflammatories 68

Recognizing the Connection Between Inflammation and Diet: 68

Foods to Steer Clear of That Cause Inflammation: 69
Refined Carbohydrates: 70
Trans Fats 70
Saturated Fats 71
Anti-Inflammatory Herbs and Cooking Methods: 71
Using Heart-Healthy Oils 71
Adding Herbs and Spices 72
Try These Tasty Anti-Inflammatory Recipes: 72
Turmeric-Ginger Lentil Soup 72
Avocado and Kale Quinoa Salad 73
Omega-3 Fatty Acids in the Diet for Joint Health 73
CHAPTER SEVEN 76
Techniques for Eating Out 76
Confidently Navigating Restaurant Menus 76
When Dining Out, Make the Correct Inquiries 77
Advice on How to Socialise Without Losing Your Diet 78

Travel Advice for Sticking to Your
Dietary Objectives 79

Modifications to Lifestyle to Reduce GERD
Symptoms 81

    Dietary changes: 81

    Eating habits: 82

    Weight control: 82

    Quitting smoking: 82

    Techniques for Reducing Stress and
    Unwinding 83

    Including Exercise to Promote Digestive
    Health: 84

CHAPTER EIGHT 86

Monitoring Symptoms and Development for
the Best Possible Care 86

Special Recommendations for Individuals
with Diabetes 87

Blood Sugar Regulation Is Critical for
GERD Management: 88

Low-Carb Strategies for GERD-Affected
Diabetics: 89

Diabetes-Compatible Recipes & Dinner
Suggestions: 90

Effective Blood Sugar Level Monitoring
.... 90

CHAPTER NINE 92
FAQs and Common Questions 92
Taking Care of Weight Management Concerns 92
Handling Acid Reflux After Dark: 94
How to Handle GERD Flare-Ups: 95
Frequently Asked Questions Regarding Diet and GERD Management: 99
Lentil and vegetable soup 103
Baked Chicken with Asparagus and Sweet Potatoes: 104
THE END 112

© 2024 Dr. Shayla Lewis All rights reserved.

No part of this publication may be reproduced, distributed, or transmitted in any form or by any means, including photocopying, recording, or other electronic or mechanical methods, without the prior written permission of the publisher, except in the case of brief quotations embodied in critical reviews and certain other noncommercial uses permitted by copyright law.

DISCLAIMER

Write a brief complete Disclaimer for my diet cook book telling them that the author is not in any association with any company, business or individual and also this book is written by the authors knowledge and understanding

The information provided in this diet cookbook is based on the author's personal knowledge and understanding. The author is not affiliated with, endorsed by, or associated with any company, business, or individual. The recipes and dietary advice contained within this book are intended for informational purposes only. Readers should consult with a healthcare professional or a registered dietitian before making any significant changes to their diet or lifestyle. The author assumes no responsibility for any adverse effects

CHAPTER ONE

An explanation of acid reflux disease (GERD)

Acid reflux from the stomach frequently flows back into the esophagus due to Gastrointestinal Reflux Disease (GERD), a chronic condition that can be uncomfortable and potentially harm the lining of the esophagus. Gaining an understanding of the underlying causes, symptoms, and potential complications of GERD is essential.

The lower esophageal sphincter (LES), a muscle ring that seals the opening between the esophagus and stomach and keeps food from going backward, is the main cause of gastroesophageal reflux disease (GERD). It can weaken or malfunction. Stomach acid can reflux into the esophagus when this sphincter relaxes improperly or weakens, causing irritation, inflammation, and a range of symptoms including heartburn, regurgitation, chest pain, and trouble swallowing.

Obesity, hiatal hernias, certain drugs, smoking, and dietary practices are among the factors that might lead to GERD. Evaluation of symptoms, medical history, and diagnostic procedures like endoscopy or pH monitoring are frequently combined to provide a diagnosis.

Diet is Important for GERD Management

To control GERD symptoms and avoid flare-ups, diet is essential. While some meals and beverages might help ease discomfort and encourage healing, others can exacerbate symptoms of acid reflux or cause it to flare again.

Important food factors for managing GERD include:

Foods Known to Trigger Acid Reflux: Acid reflux is known to be triggered by high-fat, spicy, caffeine, alcohol, citrus fruits, tomatoes, and fizzy drinks. These foods should be avoided or kept to a minimum.

Control Your Portion: Eating too much might strain the stomach and make GERD symptoms worse. Reflux episodes might be less common by eating smaller, more frequent

Eating Slowly: Bloating and reflux can be exacerbated by swallowing too much air, which can be avoided by chewing food completely and taking your time.

Sustaining a Healthy Weight: Being overweight, particularly in the abdominal area, can raise blood pressure in the belly and exacerbate GERD symptoms. Maintaining a healthy weight and reducing symptoms can be achieved by eating a balanced diet and exercising frequently.

Selecting GERD-Friendly Foods: People with GERD may usually handle lean meats, whole grains, fruits, vegetables (apart from those that provoke symptoms), non-acidic drinks like water, herbal tea, and low-fat dairy products.

Meal Timing: You can lower your risk of reflux at night by eating at least two to three hours before you lay down or go to bed.

Hydration: Throughout the day, sipping lots of water aids in promoting healthy digestion by reducing stomach acid.

Through thoughtful food selection and the inclusion of GERD-friendly foods in regular meals, people can enhance their quality of life and effectively control their symptoms.

The Fundamentals of Antioxidant-Rich, Low-Carb, and Anti-Inflammatory Diets

By lowering inflammation, enhancing digestive health, and enhancing general well-being, low-carb, antioxidant-rich, and anti-inflammatory diets may be beneficial for people with GERD.

Low-Carb Diet: Cutting back on carbs, especially refined sweets and grains, will help your blood sugar stay stable and lessen the frequency with which you experience GERD symptoms. Sustained energy can be obtained without inducing reflux by placing an emphasis on lean meats, healthy fats, and non-starchy veggies.

Antioxidant-Rich Diet: Oxidative stress and inflammation are linked to the pathophysiology of GERD and can be countered by antioxidants. Antioxidant-rich foods like berries, leafy greens, nuts, seeds, and vibrant fruits and vegetables can help shield the lining of the esophagus and lessen the symptoms of GERD.

Anti-Inflammatory Diet: The onset and course of GERD are significantly influenced by chronic inflammation. Whole foods, omega-3 fatty acids, turmeric, ginger, and green tea are all components of an anti-inflammatory diet that can help lessen inflammation and lessen the intensity of GERD symptoms.

Individuals with GERD may experience less discomfort, less inflammation, and better overall health results if they incorporate these dietary guidelines into their meal plans.

Managing Neuropathy and Nerve Pain

The treatment of GERD may be made more difficult by nerve discomfort and neuropathy, which can worsen digestive symptoms and lower quality of life. Creating successful treatment plans requires an understanding of how GERD and nerve pain interact.

Planning Meals and Cooking in Bulk

Meal planning's advantages for managing GERD

When it comes to treating Gastrointestinal Reflux Disease (GERD), meal planning is essential because it enables people to choose foods that are less likely to cause symptoms like heartburn, acid reflux, and discomfort. The following are some main advantages:

Managed Portions: By organizing meals ahead of time, people can manage their portion sizes and avoid overindulging, which frequently exacerbates GERD symptoms.

Balanced Nutrition: By organizing their meals, people may make sure they are consuming the right amount of fiber, vitamins, and minerals, all of which can improve digestive health and lessen the intensity of GERD symptoms.

Avoidance of Trigger Meals: People can prevent their GERD symptoms by carefully choosing ingredients and recipes that don't include meals like caffeine, spicy or acidic foods, or fatty or greasy foods.

Consistent Eating pattern: Meal planning can assist create a regular eating pattern that will help control digestion and lessen the chance of acid reflux attacks.

Cost-effective: By minimizing food waste and avoiding impulsive takeaway or dining out, which may include more costly and possibly triggering foods, meal planning can help people save money.

CHAPTER TWO

A Comprehensive Guide for Meal Planning:

Determine Your Dietary Restrictions and Needs: Take into account any foods that make your GERD symptoms worse when determining your dietary needs. If you need specific guidance, speak with a dietician or healthcare professional.

Make a Menu: **Arrange your meals for the coming week, making sure to include a range of GERD-friendly foods including whole grains, lean proteins, fruits, veggies, and low-fat dairy. To maintain meal interest, strive for a harmony of flavors and textures.**

Make a Shopping List: **Make a list of the ingredients you'll need for the coming week based on your menu. Follow your list to prevent making impulsive purchases of trigger foods.**

Prepare Ingredients: Allocate time for prepping ingredients, like chopping veggies, marinating meats, and boiling grains. This will expedite the cooking process and save time on hectic weekdays.

Cook in Batches: Prepare bigger batches of food that can be divided into portions and kept in the fridge for later use. Those with hectic schedules who might not have time to cook every day would find this very useful.

Store Correctly: To keep prepared meals and ingredients fresh and safe to eat, store them in airtight containers or freezer bags. For simple identification, label containers with the contents and the date.

Recommendations for Busy People on Batch Cooking:

Select Time-Efficient Recipes: Go for dishes like casseroles, soups, stews, and stir-fries that are simple to make in big quantities and quick to put together.

Invest in Top-Rated Storage Containers: For easy meal preparation and reheating, make an investment in top-notch storage containers that are safe to use in the microwave and freezer.

Use Kitchen Appliances: To expedite batch cooking and reduce hands-on cooking time, make use of kitchen appliances such as sheet pans, pressure cookers, and slow cookers.

Prepare Ahead: Allocate a specific period each week for meal preparation and bulk cooking. You'll maintain organization and make sure you have wholesome meals available all week long if you do this.

Rotate Meals: Spread out your batch-cooked meals throughout the week to prevent meal wear. Vary up the flavors and ingredients to keep things fresh.

Convenient Storage and Freezing Methods:

Portion Control: To make it simpler to grab and reheat meals as needed, divide batch-cooked dishes into individual or family-sized portions before storing them.

Freeze Meals Correctly: To preserve quality and avoid freezer burn, wrap and label meals correctly before freezing. To avoid ice crystals forming, use freezer-safe containers or bags and press out as much air as you can.

Use Freezer-Friendly items: To guarantee the best texture and flavor when reheated, select items that freeze well, such as cooked grains, beans, soups, and sauces.

Safely Thaw: To prevent bacterial growth and preserve food safety, thaw frozen meals in the refrigerator for the entire night or by using your microwave's defrost setting.

Example Menus for Various Dietary Choices:

Low-Acid Dietary Schedule:

Muesli with sliced bananas and almond milk for breakfast.

Lunch consists of grilled chicken salad dressed with cucumbers, mixed greens, and balsamic vinaigrette.

Steamed broccoli and baked salmon served with quinoa for dinner.

Meal Plan for Vegetarians:

Greek yogurt parfait with mixed berries and oats for breakfast.

Lentil and vegetable soup served with whole grain toast for lunch.

Dinner is marinara sauce, whole wheat pasta, and eggplant parmesan.

Whole Wheat Meal Plan:

Gluten-free bread and scrambled eggs with spinach for breakfast.

Quinoa salad with roasted veggies and a dressing made of lemon and tahini for lunch.

Dinner consists of roasted asparagus, quinoa pilaf, and grilled prawns.

These batch cooking and meal planning techniques let people enjoy a range of tasty and nourishing meals while successfully managing their GERD symptoms. It's critical to pay attention to your body and modify your diet plan as necessary to discover what suits you the best.

Nerve pain and neuropathy can affect numerous sections of the body, including the digestive system, and present in a variety of ways, such as tingling, burning, stabbing, and numbness. The gastrointestinal tract's regular operation may occasionally be interfered with by nerve injury or dysfunction, resulting in symptoms like dysmotility, visceral hypersensitivity, and altered pain perception.

In people with GERD, several conditions can lead to nerve discomfort and neuropathy, such as:

Chronic Acid Exposure: **Extended exposure to stomach acid in the esophagus might worsen neuropathic pain by irritating nerve endings.**

Inflammation: **GERD-related inflammatory processes have the potential to exacerbate nerve fiber sensitivity and exacerbate neuropathic pain.**

Side effects of medicine: **Proton pump inhibitors (PPIs), a class of medication used to treat GERD symptoms, have the potential to cause neurotoxicity and worsen neuropathic pain.**

Nutritional Deficiencies: Nerve damage and neuropathic symptoms can result from deficiencies in vital nutrients, such as vitamin B12, folate, and magnesium, which are common in GERD patients owing to malabsorption or dietary limitations.

In the context of GERD, managing nerve pain and neuropathy necessitates a multimodal strategy that includes:

Optimising GERD Treatment: Acid reflux and nerve sensitivity can be lessened by successfully controlling GERD symptoms through dietary adjustments, lifestyle changes, and medication adherence.

Pain Management treatments: Neuropathic pain can be reduced and quality of life enhanced by utilizing pain management treatments such as pharmaceutical therapy, physical therapy, acupuncture, and nerve blocks.

Resolving Nutritional Deficiencies: Reducing neuropathic symptoms and promoting nerve health can be achieved by identifying and addressing nutritional deficiencies through dietary changes or supplements.

Stress Management: You can lessen nerve discomfort and encourage relaxation by engaging in stress-reduction practices including progressive muscle relaxation, deep breathing exercises, and mindfulness meditation.

Through the implementation of comprehensive treatment strategies and the resolution of underlying causes causing nerve pain and neuropathy in GERD patients, healthcare practitioners can optimize patient outcomes and improve symptom management.

Adopting a Healthful Lifestyle for Prolonged Well-Being

For GERD sufferers to maximize symptom control, avoid problems, and advance long-term wellness, they must adopt a healthy lifestyle. Making different lifestyle adjustments can help people take charge of their health and enhance their general quality of life.

CHAPTER THREE

Important elements of a GERD sufferer's healthy lifestyle include

Dietary Modifications: Reducing reflux symptoms and supporting digestive health can be achieved by implementing a GERD-friendly diet that emphasizes whole, nutrient-dense foods, limiting trigger foods, and encouraging appropriate portion control.

Frequent Exercise: Maintaining a healthy weight, enhancing gastrointestinal motility, and lowering stress levels are all benefits of frequent exercise, which includes walking, cycling, swimming, or yoga. These factors all assist control of GERD.

Stress Management: You can lessen psychological stress by engaging in stress-reduction practices including progressive muscle relaxation, deep breathing exercises, meditation, and time spent in nature.

An explanation of acid reflux disease (GERD)

Acid reflux from the stomach frequently flows back into the esophagus due to Gastrointestinal Reflux Disease (GERD), a chronic condition that can be uncomfortable and potentially harm the lining of the esophagus. Gaining an understanding of the underlying causes, symptoms, and potential complications of GERD is essential.

The lower esophageal sphincter (LES), a muscle ring that seals the opening between the esophagus and stomach and keeps food from going backward, is the main cause of gastroesophageal reflux disease (GERD). It can weaken or malfunction. Stomach acid can reflux into the esophagus when this sphincter relaxes improperly or weakens, causing irritation, inflammation, and a range of symptoms including heartburn, regurgitation, chest pain, and trouble swallowing.

Obesity, hiatal hernias, certain drugs, smoking, and dietary practices are among the factors that might lead to GERD. Evaluation of symptoms, medical history, and diagnostic procedures like endoscopy or pH monitoring are frequently combined to provide a diagnosis.

Diet is Important for GERD Management

To control GERD symptoms and avoid flare-ups, diet is essential. While some meals and beverages might help ease discomfort and encourage healing, others can exacerbate symptoms of acid reflux or cause it to flare again.

Important food factors for managing GERD include:

Foods Known to Trigger Acid Reflux: Acid reflux is known to be triggered by high-fat, spicy, caffeine, alcohol, citrus fruits, tomatoes, and fizzy drinks. These foods should be avoided or kept to a minimum.

Control Your Portion: Eating too much might strain the stomach and make GERD symptoms worse. Reflux episodes might be less common by eating smaller, more frequent meals.

Eating Slowly: Bloating and reflux can be exacerbated by swallowing too much air, which can be avoided by chewing food completely and taking your time.

Sustaining a Healthy Weight: Being overweight, particularly in the abdominal area, can raise blood pressure in the belly and exacerbate GERD symptoms. Maintaining a healthy weight and reducing symptoms can be achieved by eating a balanced diet and exercising frequently.

Selecting GERD-Friendly Foods: People with GERD may usually handle lean meats, whole grains, fruits, vegetables (apart from those that provoke symptoms), non-acidic drinks like water, herbal tea, and low-fat dairy products.

Meal Timing: You can lower your risk of reflux at night by eating at least two to three hours before you lay down or go to bed.

Hydration: Throughout the day, sipping lots of water aids in promoting healthy digestion by reducing stomach acid.

Through thoughtful food selection and the inclusion of GERD-friendly foods in regular meals, people can enhance their quality of life and effectively control their symptoms.

The Fundamentals of Antioxidant-Rich, Low-Carb, and Anti-Inflammatory Diets

By lowering inflammation, enhancing digestive health, and enhancing general well-being, low-carb, antioxidant-rich, and anti-inflammatory diets may be beneficial for people with GERD.

Low-Carb Diet: Cutting back on carbs, especially refined sweets and grains, will help your blood sugar stay stable and lessen the frequency with which you experience GERD symptoms. Sustained energy can be obtained without inducing reflux by placing an emphasis on lean meats, healthy fats, and non-starchy veggies.

Antioxidant-Rich Diet: Oxidative stress and inflammation are linked to the pathophysiology of GERD and can be countered by antioxidants. Antioxidant-rich foods like berries, leafy greens, nuts, seeds, and vibrant fruits and vegetables can help shield the lining of the esophagus and lessen the symptoms of GERD.

Anti-Inflammatory Diet: The onset and course of GERD are significantly influenced by chronic inflammation. Whole foods, omega-3 fatty acids, turmeric, ginger, and green tea are all components of an anti-inflammatory diet that can help lessen inflammation and lessen the intensity of GERD symptoms.

Individuals with GERD may experience less discomfort, less inflammation, and better overall health results if they incorporate these dietary guidelines into their meal plans.

Managing Neuropathy and Nerve Pain

The treatment of GERD may be made more difficult by nerve discomfort and neuropathy, which can worsen digestive symptoms and lower quality of life. Creating successful treatment plans requires an understanding of how GERD and nerve pain interact.

Nerve pain and neuropathy can affect numerous sections of the body, including the digestive system, and present in a variety of ways, such as tingling, burning, stabbing, and numbness.

The gastrointestinal tract's regular operation may occasionally be interfered with by nerve injury or dysfunction, resulting in symptoms like dysmotility, visceral hypersensitivity, and altered pain perception.

In people with GERD, several conditions can lead to nerve discomfort and neuropathy, such as:

Chronic Acid Exposure: Extended exposure to stomach acid in the esophagus might worsen neuropathic pain by irritating nerve endings.

Inflammation: GERD-related inflammatory processes have the potential to exacerbate nerve fiber sensitivity and exacerbate neuropathic pain.

Side effects of medicine: Proton pump inhibitors (PPIs), a class of medication used to treat GERD symptoms, have the potential to cause neurotoxicity and worsen neuropathic pain.

Nutritional Deficiencies: Nerve damage and neuropathic symptoms can result from deficiencies in vital nutrients, such as vitamin B12, folate, and magnesium, which are common in GERD patients owing to malabsorption or dietary limitations.

In the context of GERD, managing nerve pain and neuropathy necessitates a multimodal strategy that includes:

Optimising GERD Treatment: Acid reflux and nerve sensitivity can be lessened by successfully controlling GERD symptoms through dietary adjustments, lifestyle changes, and medication adherence.

Pain Management treatments: Neuropathic pain can be reduced and quality of life enhanced by utilizing pain management treatments such as pharmaceutical therapy, physical therapy, acupuncture, and nerve blocks.

Resolving Nutritional Deficiencies: Reducing neuropathic symptoms and promoting nerve health can be achieved by identifying and addressing nutritional deficiencies through dietary changes or supplements.

Stress Management: You can lessen nerve discomfort and encourage relaxation by engaging in stress-reduction practices including progressive muscle relaxation, deep breathing exercises, and mindfulness meditation.

Through the implementation of comprehensive treatment strategies and the resolution of underlying causes causing nerve pain and neuropathy in GERD patients, healthcare practitioners can optimize patient outcomes and improve symptom management.

Adopting a Healthful Lifestyle for Prolonged Well-Being

For GERD sufferers to maximize symptom control, avoid problems, and advance long-term wellness, they must adopt a healthy lifestyle. Making different lifestyle adjustments can help people take charge of their health and enhance their general quality of life.

CHAPTER FOUR

Important elements of a GERD sufferer's healthy lifestyle include

Dietary Modifications: Reducing reflux symptoms and supporting digestive health can be achieved by implementing a GERD-friendly diet that emphasizes whole, nutrient-dense foods, limiting trigger foods, and encouraging appropriate portion control.

Frequent Exercise: Maintaining a healthy weight, enhancing gastrointestinal motility, and lowering stress levels are all benefits of frequent exercise, which includes walking, cycling, swimming, or yoga. These factors all assist control of GERD.

Stress Management: Psychological stressors that worsen GERD symptoms can be lessened by engaging in stress-reduction practices including progressive muscle relaxation, deep breathing exercises, meditation, or time spent in nature.

Sleep Hygiene: Developing healthy sleep hygiene habits can help lessen acid reflux at night and enhance the quality of your sleep overall. These habits include keeping a regular sleep schedule, establishing a calming bedtime routine, and optimizing your sleep environment.

Giving Up Smoking: Giving up smoking is essential for those who have GERD since it can weaken the lower esophageal sphincter, produce more acid, and make reflux symptoms worse.

Limiting Alcohol and Caffeine: Because both alcohol and caffeine can relax the lower esophageal sphincter and encourage the formation of acid, limiting these substances' intake can help lessen the frequency and intensity of GERD symptoms.

Long-term GERD patients can effectively control their symptoms and experience an enhanced quality of life by embracing a holistic approach to health and wellbeing that includes dietary adjustments, regular exercise, stress management, and good habits.

Fundamentals of Nutrition.
Gaining Knowledge about Micronutrients and Macronutrients

The fundamental elements of a balanced diet are macronutrients and micronutrients, each of which is important for preserving general health and well-being.

Macronutrients: These are the nutrients that the body needs in significant amounts to support different physiological processes and supply energy. Proteins, lipids, and carbs are the three main types of macronutrients. The body uses carbohydrates as its primary energy source to power bodily functions and physical activity. Proteins are necessary for the synthesis of hormones and enzymes, as well as for the maintenance and repair of tissues. Despite their frequent vilification, fats are essential for cell membrane construction, insulation, and the uptake of fat-soluble vitamins.

Micronutrients: Although they are needed in smaller quantities than macronutrients, micronutrients are just as important for preserving health. Minerals and vitamins are examples of micronutrients, and they are essential for a number of the body's biochemical activities. Vitamins like C and E, for instance, function as antioxidants and shield cells from oxidative harm. For healthy bones, muscles, and nerve transmission, minerals like calcium and magnesium are necessary.

A person can make educated dietary decisions and make sure they are getting enough nutrients by being aware of the functions of macro- and micronutrients in the body.

The Value of Protein, Fibre, and Good Fats

A balanced diet must include fiber, protein, and healthy fats, each of which has special health advantages.

Fibre: A form of carbohydrate that can be found in whole grains, fruits, vegetables, nuts, and seeds, as well as other plant-based foods. Because it gives stool more volume, encourages regular bowel movements, and lessens the likelihood of constipation, it is crucial for digestive health. Fibre is good for heart health and diabetes management since it also helps to reduce blood sugar and maintain healthy cholesterol levels.

Protein: Protein is required for the synthesis of hormones and enzymes, immune system support, and tissue growth and repair. Meat, poultry, fish, eggs, dairy products, legumes, nuts, and seeds are all excellent sources of protein. It is especially crucial for those who are physically active or trying to gain muscle mass to consume enough protein.

Healthy Fats: Including healthy fats in the diet is crucial for maintaining general health because not all fats are created equal. Foods high in monounsaturated and polyunsaturated fats, such as fatty fish, avocados, nuts, and seeds, can help lower blood pressure, reduce inflammation, and improve cognitive function. Limiting saturated and trans fats is crucial since they raise the risk of heart disease and other conditions.

People can support their best health and well-being by eating a diet high in fiber, lean protein sources, and healthy fats.

Recognising Foods and Drinks That Trigger:

For those suffering from gastrointestinal disorders like Crohn's disease, food intolerances, or irritable bowel syndrome (IBS), figuring out which foods and drinks to avoid can help control symptoms and enhance quality of life.

Trigger Foods: Foods that increase the symptoms of gastrointestinal distress, such as gas, bloating, diarrhea, or constipation, are known as trigger foods. Certain fruits and vegetables, dairy products, gluten-containing grains, spicy foods, caffeine, and alcohol are examples of common trigger foods, however, they can vary from person to person. People can find their trigger foods by keeping a food journal and observing how various foods impact their symptoms.

Trigger Beverages: Beverages, especially those heavy in carbonation, caffeine, alcohol, or artificial sweeteners, can aggravate gastrointestinal symptoms. Drinks such as coffee, tea, energy drinks, soda, and alcohol are frequently responsible for inducing gastrointestinal problems in certain people. Reducing or staying away from certain drinks could assist with symptoms and enhance digestive health in general.

People with gastrointestinal problems can enhance their quality of life and more effectively manage their symptoms by recognizing and avoiding trigger foods and beverages.

CHAPTER FIVE

Including Variation in a Balanced Diet

To provide balanced nutrition and satisfy the body's nutritional requirements, a diverse range of foods must be included in the diet.

Nutrient Diversity: Since various foods have varying amounts of nutrients, eating a broad range of foods guarantees that the body gets a varied range of vitamins, minerals, antioxidants, and other vital nutrients. Consuming a wide variety of fruits and vegetables, whole grains, lean meats, and healthy fats helps give the body the nourishment it needs to perform at its best.

Dietary Balance: A well-balanced diet consists of a combination of micronutrients (minerals and vitamins) and macronutrients (proteins, fats, and carbohydrates). Every meal should have a source of healthy fats, a serving of carbohydrates, and a source of protein.

Additionally, to optimize nutrient intake and enhance general health, give preference to whole, minimally processed foods over highly processed or refined ones.

People can make sure they are obtaining the nutrients they need for optimum health and well-being by including a range of foods in their diet.

How to Read Food Labels Expertly:

Making educated dietary decisions and choosing foods that promote health and well-being requires the ability to read food labels.

Serving Size: All of the nutrient information supplied is based on the serving size shown on the food label, so pay attention to it. Pay attention to serving sizes to prevent overindulging and to precisely monitor your intake of nutrients.

Nutrient Content: Examine the food's nutritional makeup, focusing on important elements including calories, fat (total and saturated), cholesterol, sodium, fiber, sugars, and protein. Seek foods that are low in salt, harmful fats, and added sweets and high in nutrients.

Ingredients List: Examine the list of ingredients to find out what goes into the dish. The product's most noticeable ingredients are those that are listed in descending order of weight. Select meals that have easily identifiable, basic components, and stay away from goods that have a lengthy list of artificial, preservative, and addictive substances.

For the best possible health and well-being, people can make healthier decisions and better control their diets by carefully reading and comprehending food labels.

Living Low-Carb

This chapter delves into the world of low-carb living, examining its nuances, advantages, and real-world uses for digestive health.

Examining Food Options Low in Carbs

In recent times, there has been a significant surge in the popularity of low-carb diets due to their potential health benefits and ability to help manage illnesses such as gastroesophageal reflux disease (GERD). Knowing which items fit into this nutritional plan is essential when starting a low-carb journey. Foods low in carbohydrates but high in vital nutrients including protein, fiber, healthy fats, and micronutrients are the main focus of low-carb diets. Among the best low-carb food options are:

Non-Starchy Vegetables: Asparagus, bell peppers, broccoli, cauliflower, and leafy greens are all fantastic options. They're high in fiber, vitamins, and minerals but low in carbohydrates.

Lean Proteins: Essential components of a low-carb diet include eggs, chicken, turkey, fish, tofu, and tempeh. They satisfy hunger without raising blood sugar levels and offer vital amino acids for muscle repair.

Good Fats: Nuts, seeds, avocado, coconut oil, and olive oil are good sources of fats that promote hormone synthesis and brain function while keeping you feeling full and content.

Low-Sugar Fruits: On a low-carb diet, berries including strawberries, blueberries, raspberries, and blackberries can be consumed in moderation because they have less sugar than other fruits.

Dairy: Moderate consumption of full-fat dairy products, such as Greek yogurt, cheese, and cottage cheese, is recommended. However, it's important to keep an eye out for added sugars in flavored variants.

You may maintain your gut health and build a varied and fulfilling low-carb diet plan by including these foods in your meals.

Effective Blood Sugar Management

The capacity of a low-carb diet to efficiently control blood sugar levels is one of its main benefits, particularly for those with GERD. Carbohydrates, especially refined sugars and carbs, can quickly raise and lower blood sugar levels, which can result in increased appetite, cravings, and energy swings.

People can maintain more stable blood sugar levels throughout the day by consuming fewer carbohydrates and concentrating on foods like non-starchy vegetables, lean proteins, and healthy fats that have no effect on blood sugar. Not only can this steady blood sugar regulation improve general health, but it can also help regulate GERD symptoms including better digestion and less acid reflux.

Low-Carb Diets' Advantages for GERD

Chronic acid reflux disease, or GERD, can have a serious negative effect on a person's quality of life. According to research, low-carb diets may help GERD sufferers in several ways:

Decreased Acid Reflux: Low-carb diets can help reduce reflux symptoms like heartburn and regurgitation by reducing the amount of high-carb and acidic foods that might cause reflux.

Weight control: Being overweight is frequently linked to GERD risk. Low-carb diets can help with weight loss and lower abdomen fat, which may lessen the frequency and intensity of GERD symptoms. This is especially true when combined with calorie restriction.

Improved Gut Health: By encouraging the growth of advantageous gut bacteria and lowering inflammation, low-carb diets high in fiber from non-starchy vegetables and other sources might improve gut health and potentially lessen GERD symptoms.

Balanced Blood Sugar Levels: As previously indicated, low-carb diets can assist in bringing blood sugar levels into balance. This can aid people with GERD by lowering insulin swings and encouraging improved metabolic health in general.

Yummy Low-Carb Recipes for Any Occasion
Making the switch to a low-carb diet doesn't have to mean compromising on taste or diversity in your meals. To get you started, try these delectable low-carb recipes:

Avocado and spinach omelet for breakfast, served with smoked salmon on the side.

Lunch consists of Parmesan crisps and grilled chicken Caesar salad with housemade dressing.

Dinner is grilled prawns served with pesto sauce over zucchini noodles, or zoodles.

Snacks: Cucumber slices with hummus, celery sticks with almond butter, or a handful of mixed almonds.

These meals offer vital nutrients to promote gastrointestinal health while showcasing the enjoyment and adaptability of a low-carb diet.

Advice for Eating Out While Keeping Your Carbs Low

While eating out can be difficult when on a low-carb diet, it is totally possible to maintain your nutritional objectives with a little forethought:

Examine Menus in Advance: A lot of restaurants now provide their menus online, so you may make plans in advance and choose low-carb options before you go.

Select Protein-Based Dishes: Go for meals that feature lean proteins, such as steak, fish, or grilled chicken, and serve them with salads or non-starchy vegetables.

Ask for Modifications: Don't be afraid to ask for adjustments or changes to make meals more low-carb. For example, you might ask to have extra veggies added to rice or pasta instead of rice, or you can ask to have sauces and dressings served on the side.

Be Aware of Hidden Carbs: Keep an eye out for hidden carbs in dressings, sauces, and condiments. Inquire about the ingredients or choose products that are less likely to have starches or sugars added.

5. Eat Portion Control: A lot of the time, restaurant servings are larger than they need to be. If you are dining with someone, think about splitting an entree or getting a to-go box so you can preserve half for later.

By using these suggestions, you can support your gut health objectives and maintain your low-carb lifestyle while still enjoying eating out.

Foods High in Antioxidants

Gastrointestinal reflux disease (GERD) is one disorder that affects the gastrointestinal system, which is important for our general health. When stomach acid flows back into the esophagus regularly, it can lead to GERD, which is an irritable and inflammatory condition. Effective management of GERD requires an understanding of how our diet affects the condition and how antioxidants function in it.

CHAPTER SIX
Disease of Gastrointestinal Reflux (GERD)

Heartburn, regurgitation, and difficulty swallowing are all signs of GERD, a chronic illness in which stomach acid flows back into the esophagus. This retrograde flow is typically stopped by the lower esophageal sphincter (LES), a ring of muscle at the opening between the stomach and esophagus. But with GERD, the LES may weaken or relax abnormally, which would let acid out.

GERD and Foods High in Antioxidants

Diet is a major factor in GERD management. While some meals may cause or worsen symptoms, others—especially those high in antioxidants—may help reduce pain and inflammation. Antioxidants are substances that counteract dangerous chemicals known as free radicals, which are implicated in tissue damage and inflammation.

Antioxidants' Function in Combating Inflammation

An important aspect of GERD is inflammation, which aggravates and discomforts the esophagus. By eliminating oxidative stress and scavenging free radicals, antioxidants aid in the fight against inflammation. By doing this, they aid in healing and shield the esophageal lining from harm.

Top Foods High in Antioxidants to Incorporate

Including foods high in antioxidants in your diet will help you control your GERD symptoms naturally. Among the best foods high in antioxidants are:

Berries: Anthocyanins and vitamin C, which are found in blueberries, strawberries, raspberries, and blackberries, are powerful antioxidants.

Leafy Greens: Rich in phytonutrients like lutein and zeaxanthin, as well as antioxidants like vitamins A, C, and E, spinach, kale, and Swiss chard.

Nuts and Seeds: Rich in fiber, healthy fats, and antioxidants, almonds, walnuts, flaxseeds, and chia seeds are a great source of nutrition.

Brightly colored vegetables: Beta-carotene and vitamin C are abundant antioxidants found in bell peppers, carrots, and sweet potatoes.

Herbs & Spices: Strong antioxidants with anti-inflammatory qualities can be found in turmeric, ginger, and cinnamon.

Making Luminous and High-Nutrient Meals

Adding a range of vibrant fruits, vegetables, nuts, seeds, and spices to your food guarantees that you are getting a varied intake of antioxidants and other important nutrients, in addition to adding taste and texture. To enhance gastrointestinal health and increase your consumption of antioxidants, try to arrange a rainbow of colors on your plate.

Recipes for Antioxidant Smoothies & Juices

Smoothies and juices are easy methods to add extra nutrients to your diet, especially if you include items high in antioxidants.

For a cool, antioxidant-rich drink, try combining mixtures of berries, leafy greens, nuts, seeds, and spices with a liquid base like water, coconut water, or almond milk.

How to Include Superfoods in Your Diet

Superfoods are foods high in nutrients that have several health advantages, including antioxidant capabilities. Superfoods such as cacao, goji berries, spirulina, and acai berries can provide your diet an extra boost of antioxidants and other vital nutrients to support general well-being and gastrointestinal health.

To sum up, knowing how antioxidants work to manage GERD and including foods high in antioxidants in your diet can help ease symptoms, lower inflammation, and promote gastrointestinal health.

You may optimize your diet for improved digestive health and general wellness by preparing vibrant, nutrient-dense meals, adding superfoods, and making antioxidant smoothies and juices.

Consuming Anti-Inflammatories
Recognizing the Connection Between Inflammation and Diet:

awareness of how our dietary decisions affect our general health, especially in relation to gastrointestinal (GI) health, requires an awareness of the connection between inflammation and diet. The body naturally reacts to damaging stimuli, such as infections, poisons, or injuries, by producing inflammation. On the other hand, gastrointestinal illnesses such as Crohn's disease, ulcerative colitis, and inflammatory bowel disease (IBD) might be attributed to chronic inflammation.

The body's inflammatory levels are significantly regulated by diet. Certain meals have the ability to either increase or decrease inflammation. Increased inflammation, for example, has been associated with diets heavy in processed foods, refined carbohydrates, sugar, and unhealthy fats (including trans and saturated fats). Conversely, diets high in antioxidants, good fats (such as omega-3 fatty acids), whole grains, fruits, and vegetables offer anti-inflammatory qualities.

Foods to Steer Clear of That Cause Inflammation:

In an anti-inflammatory dietary plan, a number of foods have been identified as potential triggers for inflammation and should be limited or avoided. Among them are:

Processed Foods: Added sugars, bad fats, and artificial additives are common in processed foods, and they can all lead to inflammation.

Refined Carbohydrates: Items high in sugar, such as white rice, bread, and snacks, can raise blood sugar levels and aggravate inflammation.

Sugary Drinks: Fruit juices and sodas with added sugar have been related to a number of health issues, including inflammation.

Trans Fats: Known to exacerbate inflammation and raise the risk of chronic illnesses, trans fats are included in partially hydrogenated oils, which are utilized in a lot of processed and fried meals.

Saturated Fats: Although red meat and full-fat dairy products are good sources of saturated fats, consuming significant quantities of these fats might exacerbate inflammation.

Anti-Inflammatory Herbs and Cooking Methods:

Meal preparation and cooking techniques can have an impact on the inflammatory potential of our food in addition to selecting anti-inflammatory items. Herbs and cooking methods that can help lower inflammation include:

Cooking techniques including grilling, steaming, and roasting help foods retain their nutrients without adding unnecessary fats, which makes them appropriate for an anti-inflammatory diet.

Using Heart-Healthy Oils: Use heart-healthy oils, such as olive, avocado, or coconut oil, which contain anti-inflammatory components, rather than oils high in saturated or trans fats.

Adding Herbs and Spices: A number of herbs and spices, including cinnamon, ginger, garlic, and turmeric, have strong anti-inflammatory qualities and can be added to food to improve its flavor and nutritional value.

Try These Tasty Anti-Inflammatory Recipes: It need not be difficult to prepare tasty meals that are also anti-inflammatory. You can include these delectable foods in your anti-inflammatory diet plan:

Turmeric-Ginger Lentil Soup: Packed with protein and fiber, this filling soup blends the anti-inflammatory qualities of turmeric and ginger with lentils to create a satisfying and healthy dinner.

Salmon is high in omega-3 fatty acids, which have been demonstrated to lower inflammation. Try it grilled with lemon and dill. Squeezing a lemon and adding fresh herbs like dill enhances flavor without adding bad fats.

Avocado and Kale Quinoa Salad: Quinoa is a nutrient-dense whole grain that can be the foundation of a tasty salad. For a cool and soothing dinner, toss in avocado, kale, cherry tomatoes, and a simple vinaigrette consisting of olive oil and balsamic vinegar.

Omega-3 Fatty Acids in the Diet for Joint Health:

Polyunsaturated fats, such as omega-3 fatty acids, have been demonstrated to have anti-inflammatory properties and are vital for overall health, especially when it comes to joint health. Eating more meals high in omega-3 fatty acids can help lower inflammation and ease the symptoms of rheumatoid arthritis.

Flaxseeds, chia seeds, walnuts, hemp seeds, and fatty fish including trout, salmon, mackerel, and sardines are plant-based sources of omega-3 fatty acids. Furthermore, omega-3 supplements can be taken to increase intake, particularly for individuals who may not get enough from diet alone.

Examples of these supplements are fish oil or algae oil capsules.

CHAPTER SEVEN
Techniques for Eating Out

Eating out can be difficult for people with Gastrointestinal Reflux Disease (GERD) since restaurant food frequently contains substances that can exacerbate symptoms including regurgitation, heartburn, and chest pain. Nonetheless, it is feasible to follow a GERD-friendly diet and still enjoy dining out if you have the appropriate knowledge and techniques.

Confidently Navigating Restaurant Menus

It's important to approach the menu cautiously and pay close attention to detail when dining out. Simple-to-prepare foods are ideal; stay away from foods that are highly fried, spicy, or acidic as they might aggravate GERD symptoms. Choose baked, steamed, or grilled dishes over fried ones, and inquire as to whether the chef can make your meal without adding extra sauces or spices.

Some eateries might provide a special menu item for dietary restrictions or allergies. Use this to your advantage and ask about GERD-friendly solutions. Furthermore, don't be afraid to ask the server for advice or further information on how the dishes are made.

When Dining Out, Make the Correct Inquiries

To make sure that your meal satisfies your dietary requirements, it is essential to communicate with the restaurant personnel. Ask inquiries regarding ingredients, preparation techniques, and potential substitutes when placing your order. Ask to have your food cooked with as little additional fat as possible, for instance, and find out if butter or oils are used in the cooking process.

Always err on the side of caution and choose something else if you're not sure about a specific dish or ingredient. Recall that you have the right to request adjustments to support your GERD treatment plan as an advocate for your health and well-being.

Nutritious Alternatives to Restaurant Favourites

Easy ingredient substitutions can make a lot of restaurant favorites more GERD-friendly. For instance, choose a thin-crust pizza topped with veggies and lean proteins rather than one with a thick tomato sauce and fiery pepperoni. Similarly, to control portion sizes and steer clear of extra fat and calories, request dressings and sauces on the side and go for whole grain or gluten-free options where available.

Advice on How to Socialise Without Losing Your Diet

Dining out with friends and family doesn't have to throw off your GERD treatment strategy. Think about recommending eateries that provide a range of choices, such as lighter meals and dishes that may be customized. Additionally, by striking up a discussion and savoring the company of others, concentrate on the social side of dining rather than just the food.

Offer to bring a meal that satisfies your dietary requirements if you're attending an event where food is provided. This guarantees that you'll be able to share tasty and nourishing food with others and also have something safe to eat.

Travel Advice for Sticking to Your Dietary Objectives

Travelling can provide particular difficulties for people with GERD, particularly when it comes to figuring out new foods and dining settings. Investigate local eateries that accommodate GERD-friendly menu items or offer GERD-friendly selections prior to your trip. While traveling, keeping portable, shelf-stable foods and snacks on hand can also help fend off hunger and temptation.

If you're traveling and eating out, make sure the restaurant staff is aware of your dietary restrictions and ask for advice based on the flavors and ingredients available in the area. In case of flare-ups, think about keeping antacids or other prescription drugs with you to treat your symptoms.

Overall, eating out may be enjoyed while properly treating GERD if it is planned for, communicated with, and flexible. You can confidently read restaurant menus and stick to your nutritional objectives even when traveling or interacting with others if you make educated decisions and take responsibility for your health.

Chapter 8: Handling the Symptoms of GERD

The symptoms of Gastrointestinal Reflux Disease (GERD), a chronic illness, include heartburn, regurgitation, chest pain, and difficulty swallowing. The ailment is caused by the reflux of stomach contents into the esophagus. Although medicine is an important part of managing GERD, lifestyle changes are just as important for long-term treatment and symptom relief. This chapter explores a number of effective GERD symptom treatment options, such as stress management, physical activity, herbal therapies, and symptom tracking, among others.

Modifications to Lifestyle to Reduce GERD Symptoms

Dietary changes: Some meals and drinks might relax the lower esophageal sphincter (LES) or increase the production of gastric acid, which can aggravate the symptoms of GERD. Patients are frequently told to stay away from acidic (citrus fruits, for example), fatty, spicy, caffeine-containing, chocolate-covered, and alcoholic meals. Rather, individuals are urged to increase their intake of alkaline foods such as whole grains, vegetables, lean meats, and non-citrus fruits.

Eating habits: **GERD symptoms might be made worse by eating large meals or by lying down right away afterward. Smaller, more frequent meals are preferable for patients, as is staying away from eating at least two to three hours before going to bed. Reflux during the night can also be avoided by raising the head of the bed.**

Weight control: **Carrying too much weight might strain the abdomen and cause more acid attacks. For this reason, controlling GERD requires reaching and keeping a healthy weight through diet and exercise.**

Quitting smoking: **Smoking weakens the LES and increases the production of stomach acid. Giving up smoking can greatly improve general health and lessen GERD symptoms.**

Techniques for Reducing Stress and Unwinding:

There are several ways in which stress and worry can exacerbate the symptoms of GERD, including by producing more acid and changing the motility of the gastrointestinal tract. Therefore, managing GERD requires implementing stress-reduction strategies into daily living.

Deep breathing techniques, progressive muscle relaxation, and meditation are examples of mindfulness practices that can help lower stress levels and increase relaxation, which will lessen the symptoms of GERD.

By treating the underlying psychological causes of stress and anxiety, stress-reduction methods like yoga and tai chi as well as cognitive-behavioral therapy (CBT) have also demonstrated promise in the management of GERD symptoms.

Including Exercise to Promote Digestive Health:

Frequent exercise has been linked to fewer GERD symptoms and better gastrointestinal motility. Exercise lowers stress levels, supports general well-being, and aids in maintaining a healthy weight.

For those who have GERD, low-impact workouts like cycling, walking, and swimming are especially helpful because high-impact activities can make symptoms worse.

But since it raises the danger of reflux, it's imperative to avoid doing strenuous exercise just after eating. Instead, try to get in at least 30 minutes of moderate-intensity exercise most days of the week.

Supplements and Herbal Remedies for Symptom Relief:

Although medicine and lifestyle changes are the main treatments for GERD, some people may benefit from extra symptom alleviation from herbal therapies and supplements.

In the past, people have utilized herbs like marshmallow root, ginger, licorice, and chamomile to treat digestive discomfort and possibly even GERD symptoms.

Probiotics, melatonin, and deglycyrrhizinated licorice (DGL) are a few supplements that may help treat GERD by lowering inflammation and enhancing gastrointestinal health.

Before adding any herbal remedies or supplements to your GERD treatment plan, you should speak with a healthcare provider because they can worsen underlying issues or interfere with medicine.

CHAPTER EIGHT
Monitoring Symptoms and Development for the Best Possible Care

Maintaining a symptom journal can be very helpful in figuring out the patterns and triggers related to GERD symptoms. To identify what causes their symptoms to worsen or improve, patients should keep a journal of their daily food intake, activities, stress levels, and the intensity of their symptoms.

Patients and medical professionals can evaluate the efficacy of therapy initiatives and make necessary adjustments by monitoring symptoms over time. Additionally, it encourages improved communication between the patient and their healthcare team and gives patients the confidence to actively manage their illness.

Furthermore, by keeping track of development through routine follow-up visits, medical professionals can offer patients continued support and direction, resulting in the best possible treatment for GERD and an enhanced quality of life.

Special Recommendations for Individuals with Diabetes

Recognizing the Link Between Diabetes and GERD:

Diabetes and GERD have a complicated interaction. According to research, people with diabetes have a higher risk of developing gastric reflux disease (GERD) for a number of reasons, including decreased gastroparesis, elevated abdominal pressure from obesity or insulin resistance, and changes in the lower esophageal sphincter's (LES) ability to keep stomach acid from backing up into the esophagus.

Furthermore, because of shared risk factors like obesity, a poor diet, and a sedentary lifestyle, both illnesses frequently coexist. It is essential to comprehend this relationship in order to manage both illnesses concurrently.

Blood Sugar Regulation Is Critical for GERD Management:

Controlling blood sugar is essential for the management of GERD in diabetics. Because high blood sugar interferes with the LES's ability to function and delays the emptying of the stomach, it can worsen the symptoms of GERD by increasing acid reflux.

Uncontrolled diabetes can also lead to consequences like neuropathy, which can worsen GERD symptoms by preventing the esophagus from functioning normally. Therefore, the key to effectively managing GERD in diabetics is to maintain appropriate blood sugar levels by medication, diet, and lifestyle adjustments.

Low-Carb Strategies for GERD-Affected Diabetics:

Because low-carb diets can effectively control blood sugar levels, they have become more and more popular among diabetics. In a similar vein, cutting back on carbohydrates can help those with GERD by lessening the frequency and intensity of acid reflux attacks.

Increased acid production and GERD symptoms have been related to carbohydrates, particularly refined sugars and starches. Lean proteins, healthy fats, non-starchy veggies, and low-sugar fruits are examples of whole, unprocessed foods that can help people with diabetes and GERD better control their symptoms while keeping stable blood sugar levels. Minimize your intake of carbohydrates.

Diabetes-Compatible Recipes & Dinner Suggestions:

Though it can be difficult, developing GERD-friendly dishes that are also diabetes-friendly is not impossible. It's important to include foods strong in fiber, lean proteins, and healthy fats while avoiding refined carbohydrates and added sugars.

Turkey lettuce wraps with hummus, stir-fried veggies with tofu, quinoa salad with mixed greens and avocado, and grilled salmon with roasted vegetables are a few lunch choices. Desserts can be dark chocolate covered in almond butter, chia seed pudding, or sugar-free yogurt with berries.

Effective Blood Sugar Level Monitoring:

It is imperative for patients with diabetes to regularly monitor their blood sugar levels in order to maintain maximum control and avoid complications. Continuous glucose monitoring (CGM) systems and glucometers can be used to monitor blood sugar levels throughout the day and spot trends that might influence GERD symptoms.

Blood sugar levels should be checked before and after meals, particularly when experimenting with new foods or recipes that may affect blood sugar levels and GERD symptoms. People with diabetes can more effectively manage their diabetes and GERD symptoms by being watchful and proactive in controlling their blood sugar levels.

CHAPTER NINE
FAQs and Common Questions

Taking Care of Weight Management Concerns:

Since being overweight can make acid reflux symptoms worse, managing one's weight is essential to treating GERD. We'll discuss methods for reaching and keeping a healthy weight in this part in order to reduce GERD symptoms.

It's critical to keep a healthy weight in order to manage GERD. Being overweight can put a strain on the stomach, which can cause stomach acid to reflux into the esophagus and exacerbate the symptoms of GERD. Thus, maintaining a healthy weight requires a balanced diet and consistent exercise.

You can feel full with fewer calories by increasing the amount of complete foods in your diet, such as fruits, vegetables, whole grains, and lean meats. Reducing the intake of processed meals and sugary drinks rich in calories can help with weight loss.

Controlling portions is also essential for weight management. Smaller, more frequent meals spread out throughout the day help avoid overindulging and lessen the chance of causing acid reflux attacks.

Frequent exercise not only promotes healthy weight loss but also improves digestion and lowers stress levels, both of which can exacerbate GERD symptoms. Most days of the week, try to get in at least 30 minutes of moderate-intensity activity, such as cycling, brisk walking, or swimming.

A certified dietician or another healthcare expert can offer you individualized advice on weight management techniques that are catered to your unique requirements and preferences.

Handling Acid Reflux After Dark:

Nocturnal GERD, or nighttime acid reflux, can seriously impair quality of life and interfere with sleep. This section will provide methods and advice for controlling acid reflux symptoms at night in order to encourage sound sleep.

Stomach acid reflux into the esophagus when lying down can be avoided by elevating the head of the bed with blocks or by using a wedge cushion. Reflux is less likely because of this elevation, which keeps the stomach's contents below the esophageal level.

Minimizing acid reflux at night can also be achieved by avoiding heavy meals and spicy or acidic foods in the evening. Rather, choose lighter, easier-to-digest meals that are less likely to cause discomfort.

Before resting down, make sure you give your body enough time to digest. To ensure that your stomach has enough time to empty, try to complete meals two or three hours before going to bed.

Deep breathing, meditation, or mild yoga are examples of relaxation techniques that can be used before bed to help lower stress and improve the quality of your sleep, which may help ease the symptoms of acid reflux at night.

If these remedies don't relieve acid reflux at night, it's critical to speak with a healthcare provider to learn about other choices for therapy, such as medication or lifestyle changes.

How to Handle GERD Flare-Ups:

Although GERD flare-ups can be upsetting and distressing, there are things you can do to control your symptoms and stop them from happening again. We'll talk about helpful

GERD flare-up coping mechanisms in this part.

The secret to avoiding GERD flare-ups is knowing what foods and drinks trigger you. Foods that are spicy, citrus fruits, tomatoes, caffeine, alcohol, and fatty or fried foods are common triggers. By keeping a diet journal, you can identify the items that make your symptoms worse so you can steer clear of them going forward.

Smaller, more frequent meals might lessen the chance of overfeeding the stomach and acid episodes. In order to promote healthy digestion and reduce pressure on the lower esophageal sphincter (LES), it's also critical to chew food well and eat slowly.

Keeping up a healthy weight with diet and exercise can also help stop flare-ups of GERD. Being overweight increases the risk of acid reflux by putting pressure on the abdomen.

After eating, try not to lie down or bend over right away to avoid refluxing stomach acid into the esophagus. Rather, after eating, stay upright for two to three hours to let gravity help with digestion.

Stress-reduction methods like yoga, meditation, and deep breathing can be included in your daily routine to help reduce anxiety and lessen the chance of GERD flare-ups brought on by stress.

It's critical to speak with a healthcare provider for additional assessment and treatment options if GERD symptoms continue or get worse after taking these precautions.

Advice for Handling GERD While Expecting:

Pregnancy-related GERD symptoms are common because of hormonal changes and increased abdominal pressure. We'll look at various methods and advice for efficiently managing GERD during pregnancy in this section.

Smaller, more frequent meals spread out throughout the day might lessen the chance of acid reflux and assist avoid overloading the stomach. Reducing dietary triggers like hot, acidic, or fatty foods might also aid in discomfort relief.

To stop stomach acid from running back into the esophagus, it's critical to eat with proper posture and refrain from lying down very away after meals. To help with digestion, instead, stay upright for two to three hours after eating.

During pregnancy, raising the head of the bed using blocks or a wedge pillow can help lessen symptoms of acid reflux at night. Another way to reduce stomach strain and avoid reflux is to sleep on your left side.

Stress-reduction methods like deep breathing, meditation, or prenatal yoga can be included in your daily routine to help reduce anxiety and lessen the chance that stress will cause flare-ups of GERD.

For individualized advice and safe treatment choices for you and your unborn child, it's critical to speak with a healthcare provider if your GERD symptoms worsen or continue throughout your pregnancy.

Frequently Asked Questions Regarding Diet and GERD Management:

We'll address some frequently asked questions and issues about controlling GERD with dietary and lifestyle changes in this section.

Can GERD symptoms be brought on by specific foods? A: It's true that some foods and drinks might make GERD symptoms worse. Foods that are spicy, acidic (like citrus fruits and tomatoes), fried or greasy, caffeine, alcohol, and carbonated drinks are common triggers. Food diaries can be a useful tool for identifying triggers and helping you stay away from them in the future.

Are there any changes you can make to your lifestyle to assist ease the symptoms of GERD? A number of lifestyle changes can indeed help reduce GERD symptoms. These include eating smaller, more frequent meals, avoiding lying down right afterward, raising the head of the bed, steering clear of trigger foods, and engaging in stress-reduction exercises like meditation or deep breathing.

Is it possible to control GERD symptoms with medication? A: It is true that drugs like antacids, H2 receptor blockers, and proton pump inhibitors (PPIs) can lessen the production of stomach acid and ease the symptoms of GERD. Before beginning any drug, you should, however, speak with a healthcare provider to establish the best course of action for your particular needs and medical background.

Is it okay to take over-the-counter antacids when expecting? A: While some over-the-counter antacids are thought to be safe to take while pregnant, it's imperative to speak with a doctor before taking any medicine, including antacids. They are able to offer customized advice and suggest the safest and best courses of action for treating GERD symptoms during pregnancy.

Is it possible to treat GERD alone with dietary and lifestyle modifications? A: Although GERD symptoms can be lessened and the frequency and intensity of flare-ups can be decreased with diet and lifestyle changes, GERD is a chronic condition that may need continuous care. Working together with a healthcare provider is crucial to creating a thorough treatment plan that takes into account your unique requirements and objectives.

People can improve their quality of life by learning more about GERD management options and making educated decisions by attending to these often-asked questions and concerns.

Recipes:

Banana and almond butter with muesli:

For breakfast, try muesli with a dollop of almond butter and sliced banana on top.

Lunch consists of grilled chicken over a mixed green salad with whole grain bread on the side.

Steamed broccoli and baked salmon served with quinoa for dinner.

Snack: A handful of almonds and some apple slices.

Lentil and vegetable soup:

Whole grain bread with avocado spread for breakfast.

Lunch consists of whole grain crackers and a soup made with vegetables and lentils.

Brown rice and grilled tofu paired with roasted vegetables for dinner.

Snack: Hummus-topped carrot sticks.

Stir-fried vegetables with quinoa:

Greek yogurt topped with berries and honey for breakfast.

Quinoa and vegetable stir-fry with prawns or tofu for lunch.

Dinner is marinara-sauced turkey meatballs served over zucchini noodles.

Snack: Almond butter-topped rice cakes.

Baked Chicken with Asparagus and Sweet Potatoes:

Smoothie for breakfast consisting of almond milk, spinach, and banana.

Lunch consists of baked chicken breast, asparagus, and roasted sweet potato.

Dinner consists of steamed broccoli on the side and whole wheat spaghetti with marinara sauce.

Snack: Cucumber slices with tzatziki dressing.

Avocado and Salmon Salad Dressing:

Chia seed pudding with mixed berries for **breakfast.**

Lunch is a salad of salmon, mixed greens, avocado, and dressing made with lemon and tahini.

Dinner is brown rice and stir-fried tofu with mixed vegetables.

Snack: Peanut butter-covered celery sticks.

Stuffed bell peppers with turkey and quinoa:

Whole grain cereal, almond milk, and sliced strawberries for breakfast.

Bell peppers filled with turkey and quinoa for lunch.

Dinner is quinoa salad and grilled prawn skewers.

Snack: Avocado slices on top of rice cakes.

Curry with vegetables and chickpeas:

Smoothie bowl with spinach, mango, and coconut milk for breakfast.

Brown rice with vegetable and chickpea curry for lunch.

Dinner is wild rice, roasted Brussels sprouts, and baked fish.

Snack: Dried fruit and nuts combined in trail mix.

Lasagna with eggplant and zucchini:

Whole grain bread with tomato slices and mashed avocado for breakfast.

Lunch is lasagna made with eggplant and zucchini with a side salad.

Steamed green beans and quinoa pilaf accompanied by a grilled chicken breast for dinner.

Snack: Guacamole with sliced bell peppers.

Salad with Mediterranean Couscous:

Oats for breakfast made the night before with sliced banana and almond butter.

Mediterranean couscous salad with olives and feta cheese for lunch.

Dinner is baked cod served with couscous and roasted carrots.

Snack: Granola and Greek yogurt.

Tacos with black beans and vegetables:

Whole grain English muffins topped with spinach and scrambled eggs for breakfast.

Avocado slices with black bean and vegetable tacos for lunch.

Dinner is quinoa salad and grilled portobello mushrooms.

Snack: Cottage cheese and sliced pears.

Recipes:

Oatmeal Banana Pancakes:

A mild breakfast alternative that uses oat flour and mashed bananas, which are less prone to cause reflux.

Baked Casserole with Vegetables and Chicken:

A recipe consisting of lean chicken breast, various veggies, and a light sauce that is both comforting and GERD-friendly.

Ginger-Turmeric Soup with Carrots:

A calming soup that is ideal for relieving GERD symptoms since it contains anti-inflammatory components like ginger and turmeric.

Avocado and Salmon Salad:

A simple olive oil and lemon dressing highlights the omega-3-rich salmon and creamy avocado in this light and nutrient-dense salad.

Bell peppers stuffed with quinoa:

Packed with nutrients, these bell peppers are loaded with quinoa, veggies, and lean protein to provide a filling, reflux-friendly supper.

Lemon and Herb Baked Cod:

Mildly delicious cod fillets cooked with lemon and fresh herbs provide a mild yet satisfying seafood choice.

Salad with spinach and lentils:

A high-fiber salad made with delicate spinach leaves and protein-rich lentils dressed with a simple vinaigrette.

Stir-fried turkey with vegetables:

A flavorful stir-fry recipe with lean turkey breast strips and a variety of vibrant vegetables that are seasoned with garlic and ginger.

Sweet potatoes mashed:

Rich, creamy mashed sweet potatoes with a touch of cinnamon make a calming and wholesome side dish.

Apples Baked with Walnuts and Cinnamon:

- Warm baked apples with crisp walnuts and a dash of cinnamon make a naturally sweet and GERD-friendly dessert.

30-Dal Plan:

First Day:

Banana oat pancakes for breakfast

Snack: Melon slices

Carrot soup with ginger and turmeric for lunch

Snack: Hummus on Whole Grain Crackers

Supper is a casserole of vegetables and baked chicken.

Maintain a similar schedule throughout the month, making sure to consume a balance of fruits, vegetables, whole grains, lean proteins, and healthy fats. To maintain interest in meals and follow GERD management guidelines, include a range of flavors and textures. In order to assist reduce symptoms, counsel patients to eat smaller, more frequent meals, stay away from foods that cause symptoms, such as spicy or acidic foods, and avoid lying down right after eating.

In summary, gastrointestinal health and general well-being can greatly benefit from using an anti-inflammatory food regimen. People can support a healthy gut and lower their risk of chronic diseases linked to inflammation by learning about the connection between diet and inflammation, avoiding foods that exacerbate inflammation, utilizing anti-inflammatory cooking methods and herbs, experimenting with flavorful recipes, and including omega-3 fatty acids for joint health.

THE END

www.ingramcontent.com/pod-product-compliance
Lightning Source LLC
Chambersburg PA
CBHW052327220526
45472CB00001B/310